Alternative Healing through Chromotherapy:

A Guide to How Color Therapy Can Energize Your Life

By Lilia Seven
www.bioenergoterapeut.ro
(Maria Ciobanu)

Alternative Healing through Chromotherapy:
A Guide to How Color Therapy Can Energize Your Life

Published by Amazon.com
Copyright © 2013
All rights reserved.

Alternative Healing through Chromotherapy:
A Guide to How Color Therapy Can Energize Your Life

Table of Contents:

Introduction

A Background on How Color Affects and Heals

Chromotherapy, or *color therapy*, is a method of therapy that is done using color. In itself color does not heal, but it has been said that it enables the body to heal itself.

It probably has something to do with light, frequency, and vibration and how everything works together to make the whole. That is why color therapy is a form of *holistic healing* – it aims to see the whole picture. Colors have different frequencies and vibrations and even correspond to a certain note on the musical scale.

We have heard the words: green with envy, in the pink of health, down in the blues, red carpet treatment, and such. Since the mind and emotions are the most powerful energies on earth, people have come to associate colors with emotions and vice-versa.

In order to better understand how color affects our lives, let us see how it has evolved from the simple consciousness of early man to how we have come to use it now in our daily lives.

Humans are *a feeling species*. Before there was science, there was already feeling. There was observation. People of old had fantastic basic survival skills. It's eat or be eaten. It means having to pit against huge animals like dinosaurs. Unschooled as people may have been in the early days, we cannot really discount their ingenious contribution to the advancement we are now experiencing. They pretty much laid the foundation for the comforts and knowledge we are now enjoying.

They were great observers and appreciators of nature. These hardy people were in touch with nature, with the elements. It must have been a really tough existence with no comfort or luxury as we are enjoying right now. Theirs was *a survival consciousness*. They literally had to plant their ears on the ground and feel any unusual vibration or turbulence for that surely signaled earth movement or animal movement, consequently endangering their safety. Their ideas were astute observations about the things that happened each day as they interacted with everything around them.

The people of old were more *in touch with nature* for they lived with nature. There were no technical or mechanical gadgets like clocks, computers, conveniences, and contrivances that existed.

They lived and survived through their own basic instincts and allowed their strong powers of observation to guide them through life. Through observation, they realized green gourds and leaves were bitter, yellow citrus fruits were a bit sour and tangy, red and orange fruits were relatively sweet and pleasant, and that apart from blueberries, there were not much blue fruits at all.

Before the colors were even named, their concept of tint has already existed. They knew the color red for there was much blood when they had wars or when they hunted. There was no time to seek illumination. Their thoughts were focused on survival.

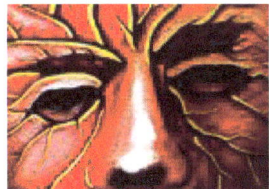 Red probably was the most basic and powerful color then, signifying blood from wars for the men and menstrual blood and childbirth for the women. The Celts and American Indians wore war paints on their faces, while other tribes like Australian aborigines honored the earth colors that were abundant in their locality by expressing them through their tribal art.

African and Arab tribes also had their own vivid colors on their faces, clothes, and homes to signify strength, courage, war, peace, intimidation, status, and protection.

European colonizers were more fascinated by trade. They were more interested in the gold they could stash or melt to add to their coffers, oftentimes, on the pretext of offering religion to the people they called "backward natives".

Of course back then when the early primitive people were *closer to the elements*, they could not verbalize what colors were and how these could affect us. But they sure could taste, identify, and differentiate what tasted good and what looked good. They made use of whatever resources they had, mostly plant- and animal-derived.

In those early days the colors that probably predominated were red, orange, yellow, black, browns, blue, white, and greens. If one were to believe in osmosis, we humans adapted and evolved and when we were intrigued by new things which we found pleasing. Surely we wanted to have more of it and, when agriculture came to the fore, we started producing more colorful and exciting foods; for with color and excitement come adventure and sophistication!

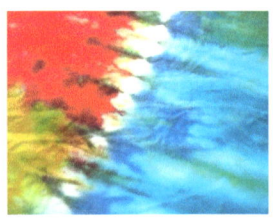 Then there was the advent of vegetable-colored dyes like the famous purple dye from Tyre meant for royalty. We started to have fashionable clothes, tapestries, and looms. Following all these materials next came the discovery and development of giant molecules which led to strong and colorful plastics. Our food had similarly become bigger, tastier, more colorful, more abundant, and lab-based. Now, looking back, we really have come a long way.

And to think that back then, our ancestors only had the sun, the moon, the stars, the clouds, and the rainbows; there was only the sky, thunder, lightning, animals, and vegetation to keep them company. Such was their focus and consciousness.

Nonetheless, *a consciousness about natural healing* already existed. Women have always been known to be healers. They started as oracles in Greece, then the midwives, virgins, and crones got into the picture as well.

It is a basic instinct for woman to heal and nurture. But I doubt it if they started color therapy for, in those early days, they healed with the scent and flavor of poultices and with the love and care they had in their hearts. They were the ones that kept the home fires burning when their warrior lords and hunters would come home from their masculine tasks.

How then did color therapy come about?

It seems the visionary Arab physician Avicenna (980-1037) was the early proponent. He saw color's vital importance in diagnosis and in treatment. He first discussed *Chromotherapy* in his work, "The Canon of Medicine".

Avicenna wrote that *color is an "observable symptom of disease".* He created a chart that related color to the temperature and physical condition of the body. He observed how red would move the blood, how blue or white cooled it, and how yellow reduced pain and inflammation.

In 1876, the American general Augustus Pleasanton published his book, "The Influence of the Blue Ray of the Sunlight and of the Blue Color of the Sky". The civil war general apparently conducted experiments and wrote in the book that the color blue can improve the growth of crops and livestock and can help heal diseases in humans.

This discovery led to modern Chromotherapy. Other famous practitioners similarly influenced were Dr. Seth Pancoast ("Light and Its Rays as Medicine") and Edwin Dwight Babbitt ("The Principles of Light and Color"). It would be worthwhile studying their works as they laced their work with color, with mysticism and spirituality – to the point of occultism.

Another color enthusiast was Hindu scientist Dinshah P. Ghadiali who claimed that *colored rays have various therapeutic effects on organisms*. He believed that colors have chemical potencies and higher octaves of vibration. He also believed that certain colors either stimulate or inhibit organs and systems.

Not everyone acknowledges the healing effects of color, especially if they have been largely schooled in science. They will demand hard proof that such therapy actually works. But then again, what may work for one may not necessarily work for another.

Sometimes a placebo works because of a person's deep faith in a particular treatment. As with everything else, it is really the mind that is both the source of pain and of healing.

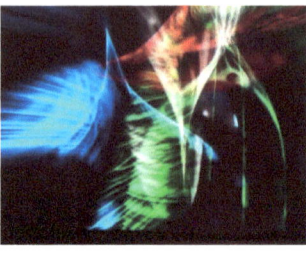

Colors vibrate at a certain frequency. There is a perfect match for what color corresponds to which organ or gland in our body. The *chakras*, our energy centers, work hand-in-hand with the endocrine system. It is this system which helps regulate our hormones and bodily functions.

You will find out in the following four (4) chapters the various *color therapy methods*, four of which are cited and explained, each with practical techniques for easy implementation.

In this Guide, you will also discover which color corresponds to which part of the body, chakra, and which color(s) can help resolve health or emotional issues in your lives. Not only will they energize you but they will also create that much-needed balance and the happiness which results. For in the end, that's really what people care about: that we become happy.

Chapter 1: Viewing the Rainbow

This method has the ability to heal and strengthen all systems of the body's energies. For this exercise to have the desired results it is to be repeated regularly, even daily if possible.

How to Apply the Rainbow Technique

There are five (5) steps to this particular method, and the proper technique can be described as follows:

Step 1:

In the first phase, you have to choose a comfortable posture whether you are standing up or sitting down. Close your eyes and breathe deeply and slowly for three times. When you exhale you are to visualize any form of tension leaving your body...

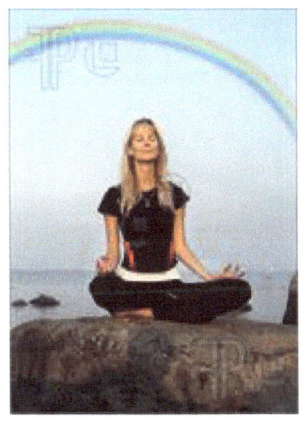

Step 2:

In the second step, you are to see in your mind's eye a rainbow that arches overhead. Follow the path of the RED light sphere that forms the lowest end of the rainbow and visualize it descending upon your head, entering your body, and emanating a red vibrating energy.

Breathe in this healing vibrant energy derived from the red spectrum of the rainbow. Let this healing energy repair and replenish any part of your body that has been weakened.

Step 3:

The third step entails your focusing on this energy and directing it towards your feet, while imagining that your whole body is enveloped with this radiant energy. See yourself shrouded with this color.

When this red vibrating energy reaches the lower legs, the red sphere dissipates its energy as it is absorbed and assimilated into your body.

Once this energy has been effectively absorbed, move on to the next color of the rainbow which is ORANGE. Using the same rainbow you were drawing from earlier, now you click on to the orange sphere from that spectrum.

Allow this orange energy vibration to fill your whole being starting from the top of your head to the tips of your toes. When this energy reaches the lower legs, this healing energy will be absorbed by the body just like in the previous red vibrating energy.

Step 4:

The fourth phase is to get every color of the rainbow as you did with the red and orange colors. That means you will be viewing the following colors in this order: RED, ORANGE, YELLOW, GREEN, BLUE, INDIGO, and PURPLE or VIOLET.

When the last color of the rainbow (purple) is absorbed you will find your whole being vibrating with energy and vitality! Your body will exhibit balance in both the physical and subtle energy fields.

Step 5:

In the last and fifth phase you will be viewing the rainbow as it arches overhead then downwards to form a circle that surrounds your body. You will discover that, at each iteration of this method, the rainbow will become stronger. At the same time, the body will become healthier and more vibrant!

Integrating all these five steps together, you now have the secret to mastering the technique of *Viewing the Rainbow*. As with everything else, practice makes perfect!

Why Viewing the Rainbow Heals

What makes viewing the rainbow so powerful and so healing?

Dr. Jacob Liberman, the "light" doctor, finds the rainbow a miracle of nature. He believes in the importance of color especially those "portions of the spectrum" that are in tune with humans.

Each color of the rainbow emits a certain vibration and frequency to which we respond and are sensitive to. Apparently, the visible spectrum we see from the beautiful and refreshing rainbow stimulates, regulates, and rebalances our body's vital functions – thus, contributing to good health, energy, and vitality.

When full-spectrum light shines into a prism, it refracts into the seven colors of the spectrum, namely: RED, ORANGE, YELLOW, GREEN, BLUE, INDIGO, and VIOLET. These are the very colors of the rainbow.

In line with the SUN'S RADIATIONS, What could be more powerful and more precise than the sun's rays which contain a whole spectrum of electromagnetic radiation that forms visible white light (full-spectrum light)?

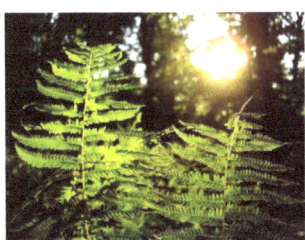

Incidentally, a single ray of sunshine contains all the colors of the spectrum. The colors that we see depend on which of the sun's rays are absorbed and which are reflected. For example we perceive the leaf to be green only because that leaf absorbs all the rays except for the color green which is reflected.

How Chakras Correlate with Colors

Chakra means spinning wheel or vortex. *Chakras* are deemed to be spiritual/energy centers and are held to be located along the spine.

Chakras or energy centers were first studied and written about some 2600 years ago. It is very interesting how our seven (7) chakras match our endocrine glands. These glands are of vital importance in the regulation of our hormones and bodily functions.

It is also fascinating to note that the chakras regulate a specific body part as well as derive their energy from the ascending colors of the rainbow.

Briefly, these colors ascend as follows:

- The *first chakra* at the base of the spine corresponds to RED.

- The *second chakra* at the lower abdomen corresponds to ORANGE.

- The *third chakra* at the solar plexus corresponds to YELLOW.

- The *fourth chakra* at the heart region corresponds to GREEN.

- The *fifth chakra* at the throat corresponds to BLUE.

- The *sixth chakra* just above the center of the brow corresponds to INDIGO.

○   Lastly, the *seventh chakra* at the crown of the
        head corresponds to VIOLET/PURPLE.

When you can see and sense the subtle connections with these
things you can only truly marvel at how light, colors, chakras, and
our bodies really need each other for continued survival.

Chapter 2: Applying Color Touch

This method is great when applied by a bioenergotherapist who
knows exactly what to do to get the desired results. His focus is
on identifying and correcting energy imbalances in a person as
exhibited on his auric field.

After careful diagnosis, he associates a specific color for a certain
disease and designs a program whereby the proper healing
energy from that color is applied to a patient.

When Color Touch Applies to Healing

Nowadays one of the most common ailments is headache which is
also one of the most easily treated through color therapy. Most
cases of migraine occur due to excessive stimulation of the *Ajna
chakra*.

The role of the Ajna chakra

Known to play a vital role in Color Touch Therapy, the Ajna chakra
has a specific location and function. It is situated at the forehead
(the third eye) and affects the pituitary gland. This is the seat of
perception and intuition. When there is an imbalance, the person

experiences undue pride, intolerance, arrogance, addiction, manipulation, and corruption.

When a migraine occurs, it merely means this chakra has been over-stimulated and one needs to cool the condition to provide relief to the patient. The bioenergotherapist will then concentrate on sending a signal or aim at projecting the energy through his hands.

Normally after a session of five minutes the results should become visible and pain will be reduced in intensity or even disappear.

<u>The colors you positively respond to</u>

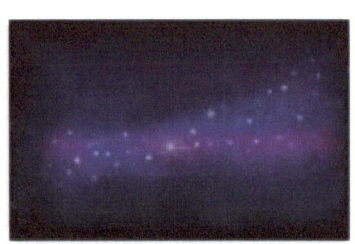

The Ajna chakra corresponds to the color INDIGO. Thus, the color to be designed in the case of headaches is to be a cold one such as PALE BLUE or a combination of BLUE and GREEN. For more intense pain, you can also use YELLOW followed by a small amount of indigo.

INDIGO is known to be the "blue-black color of the nighttime sky". The right amount of indigo will have you connected to the self, to divine wisdom, and to cosmic consciousness.

How Color Therapy Heals Migraine Headaches

Migraine sufferers notice that they experience pain when they are unwittingly exposed to glaring white light, either from intense high noon heat from the sun or from debilitating white light from fluorescent bulbs. They start sweating and their heads feel like cracking open.

When this attack happens, they become immobilized from the pain. Even their vision is temporarily affected, and they feel they cannot function at all.

The only thing to do is simply to stop whatever you are doing – all within bounds, of course. If you are working on something that may endanger your life or limb, you have to stop and take a break, excuse yourself, and find immediate relief first.

If you are feeling nauseous, you may have to find a doctor first and have your blood pressure checked, for it may signal something else.

If your blood pressure seems normal and you are not inclined to take temporary headache relief or some medication, then you can pursue Alternative Healing through Color Therapy. Here's how:

Step 1:

First, find a place where you can lie down undisturbed for a few moments. Ideally it would be in a cool, dark place, your head slightly elevated but not too much. Otherwise, you will create pressure on that sore head of yours.

Step 2:

Next, loosen any constricting clothing. Proceed to close your eyes and do some deep breathing. Instead of the usual eight counts, go for breathing in for four counts, hold, then exhale for four counts, and again, hold.

Step 3:

When you are sufficiently relaxed and you would like to seal in this healing energy derived from breathing, you can now imagine yourself being suffused by the healing blue light showering upon your head and to every part of your body.

Imagine a very light shade that you like. The color blue is anti-inflammatory, and it will cool your mind and thoughts.

Step 4:

Do this for a few minutes until you start to feel better. After the color therapy, continue lying down until you feel well enough. You can also imagine your whole body being protected by a dome of gentle white light. This is for extra protection because you will again rejoin humanity and you will be exposed to so many energies around you.

Step 5:

Sit up slowly until you get your head together, and stand up only when you are able to. Refrain from harsh, glaring lights for now.

The idea is to stop awhile, to have your blood pressure checked, to rest, to breathe slowly and properly, to fill yourself with the healing blue light, to seal in with the gentle white light, and to give yourself time to recuperate before you get back to your tasks at hand.

Chapter 3: Making Colorful Breath

To talk about this method you must first know how to breathe properly. It seems perhaps surprising to some but most people do not breathe properly. To perform correct breathing you are to breathe from the diaphragm.

Watch babies breathe when they are fast asleep and you will see how we all once breathed that way. You will see how they use their lungs and diaphragm to expand and to contract.

As we got older, we forgot this basic knowledge and started breathing differently. Thus, the cells of our body are not as nourished as they once were. And when we are afraid or tense, our breathing becomes even worse!

How to Breathe Properly Using Colored Breathing

Meditators are masters of proper breathing. They are focused on just that: *the breath* and *breathing properly* – emptying their mind and heart of all fears and erroneous thoughts.

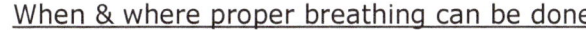

When & where proper breathing can be done

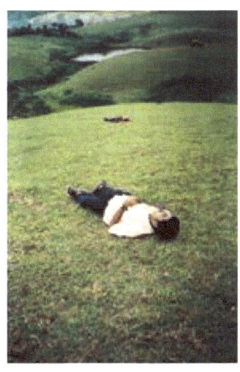

Colored breathing exercises are to be done in places where there is clean air, preferably outdoors away from polluted areas of major cities. Ideally, this is done first thing in the morning, at dawn, when the air is freshest.

If this is done accompanied by cool, mountain air, then so much the better! The oxygen from the trees will enhance the air we are breathing, and all our toxins will be absorbed by the trees.

But as most of us live in cities, we can do our morning breathing exercises in front of our windows wide open.

How to do colored breathing properly

When we do colored breathing exercises, inspired air inside the human body is converted into energy and is very much influenced by our thoughts and those of others.

It has been said that all thoughts become part of the ether and no thought is ever lost. Thus said, it would be a great idea to apply this important technique: *Focus on thinking positive thoughts that benefit all.*

One practitioner trains herself to inhale good thoughts and to exhale all negative thoughts. That being that, she cleanses herself of all forms of negativity and toxins and only takes in or breathes in that which is positive and healing.

Step 1:

In our case, let us start with proper breathing. You may do this either standing up or sitting down. Choose whatever feels more comfortable for you. The important thing is posture. Keep your spine straight and your head erect.

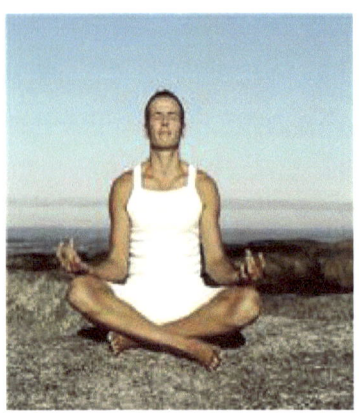

Step 2:

Breathe in air deeply from your nose. Feel your lungs expanding. Fill your lungs with good energy! Oxygen is always great for the body. It nourishes the cells of your body and clears thinking.

Step 3:

Then, gently release your breath through your mouth. With that exhalation release all the toxins from your body... Take it slow and easy. Relish the breathing process.

Here's an additional tip to successfully completing this exercise: Some meditators lie down on the floor, lower back pressed to the floor, and breathe in for a count of eight. Hold for a count of eight, then exhale for a count of eight, and hold for another count of eight. If you do this, you will find that your tummy tightens as well and that is a very good bonus!

Apart from that you also develop good posture as your lower back is pressed down on the floor. It helps release back pain as well, and it is a good overall toner for the lungs and body.

This is especially great after you feel out of sorts when you wake up in the morning. It gives you relief when you wake up with a sore or twisted back or when you feel your back is out of alignment. This floor technique always works! Combined with Reiki, this is one of the best energy healer and balancer.

Remember: *Breathing is the most basic thing and the most often overlooked.* The smartest thing to do when tired, anxious, angry, or depressed is to take a deep breath and just to focus on breathing in, breathing out, until you find some peace and calm in your persona. Only then can you act or make decisions – from this point of peace and calm.

What You Need to Know about Color and Light

You will be happy to know that the above practice on deep rhythmic breathing will help your body be receptive to color and light energies.

With these energies in mind, let's return to the seven (7) chakras which correspond to the following colors, locations, and functions. We started with this so that we may know what colors to breathe in depending on the state of our health and emotions, and so we may know what colors are needed to balance our energies.

- The *first chakra* at the base of the spine is RED and is attuned to *basic survival*.

- The *second chakra* at the lower abdomen in ORANGE and is attuned to *sexuality*.

- The *third chakra* at the solar plexus is YELLOW and is attuned to *personal power*.

- The *fourth chakra* at the heart area is GREEN and is attuned to *love*.

- The *fifth chakra* at the throat is BLUE and is attuned to *communication*.

- The *sixth chakra* just above the brow is INDIGO and is attuned to *compassion*.

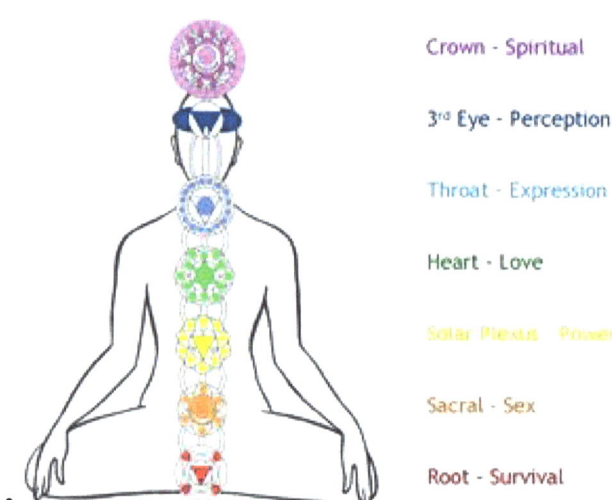

Crown - Spiritual

3rd Eye - Perception

Throat - Expression

Heart - Love

Solar Plexus - Power

Sacral - Sex

Root - Survival

- The *seventh chakra* at the crown of the head is VIOLET/PURPLE and is attuned to our *connection with the Spirit*.

Now that you are aware of deep rhythmic breathing and of the corresponding color-chakra-issues in your life and body, you need to HEAL!

All you have to do is to inhale and imagine that color enveloping your whole being. When you exhale, imagine that color blessing you from the top of your head and let it flow through your body, exiting at the feet. Allow yourself to be suffused with the color that you need, for instance:

➢ To cleanse your body of all negativity, meditate on WHITE.

➢ To heal your organs and to soothe your emotions, meditate on GREEN.

➢ To cleanse your aura, meditate on PINK.

➢ To calm yourself, meditate on BLUE.

Color therapy is helpful, but above all: *Follow your instincts and listen to your feelings. Trust yourself. Know yourself. Honor yourself.* Acknowledge your own personal emotions. This is the beginning of wisdom and of all healing – that you honor and acknowledge yourself and everything that goes on within you.

Oftentimes, the body merely exhibits the emotions we are feeling and may manifest as physical pain. When the heart hurts, you know it is not merely physiological pain but possibly because your emotions have been taken for granted. You may have been hurt by another person, or you may have allowed it as well. It always takes two.

When this happens, the only thing to do is to step back and breathe deeply, calmly, and allow clarity in the situation. More often than not we are the ones who betray ourselves and thus we feel pain. You must honor your feelings and emotions; and when you are hurting, all the more you are to be gentle with yourself.

Breathe in the color BLUE, PINK, GREEN, and INDIGO, and breathe out all the negative energy and toxins – after which, seal in all that wonderful energy with WHITE. Cocoon yourself in white light or even pink light so you may find comfort, healing, and security.

Love starts from within. Learn to love yourself first. You cannot give to others what you do not have within yourself. Similarly, you cannot give what you will not allow yourself to have. *Start with self first. Heal yourself.*

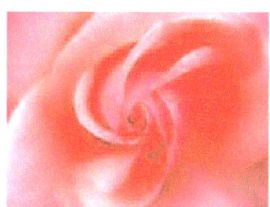 Light and color are the same. Without light, you cannot see the colors. Whether you imagine it as pink light or pink color, it's the

same. *Simply focus on the color your body needs.* Trust your instincts and be very gentle with yourself and others. That is really the secret of peace.

Chapter 4: Making Colored Chakras with Color Therapy

By now, you are aware that every color corresponds to a specific chakra and gland. In summary, you will find them listed below:

1) RED for the *Root Chakra* regulating the *Perineum*.

2) ORANGE for the *Sacral Chakra* regulating the *Suprarenal*.

3) YELLOW for the *Solar Plexus Chakra* regulating the *Lymph*.

4) GREEN for the *Heart Chakra* regulating the *Thymus*.

5) BLUE for the *Throat Chakra* regulating the *Thyroid*.

6) INDIGO for the *Third Eye Chakra* regulating the *Pineal*.

7) VIOLET for the *Crown Chakra* regulating the *Pituitary*.

To make the colored chakra, you simply have to focus on the color that calls to you based on your feelings at that moment. Then, you will know why you are drawn to that color. Your body needs that color for healing.

What Happens When You Meditate Using Color Therapy

When you meditate upon it, allowing your body to be suffused with that color – in the shade your body asks for – then you allow the chakras to spin energetically, setting the stage for healing the endocrine gland that is currently out of balance.

Everything can be done through *the mind's eye* or through *the breath*. You simply have to meditate on the color you need or to breathe in that color and you will begin to feel better and more energized!

If you are feeling low or down and out, observe what colors, food,

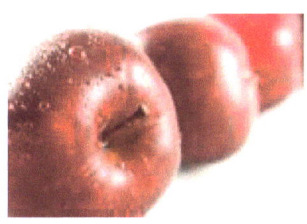 or stimulation you are drawn to. In all likelihood, that is the very color and chakra your body needs. People with low energy could be easily nurtured and nourished by a red apple that imparts its tangy juices. Even the process of biting into its crispness can awaken crispness in us, and we begin to feel better and more energized.

Nature is the great healer. The red color from the apple addresses our low energy and aids in our survival; thus, it honors the root chakra.

Nature was designed perfectly to serve the needs of man. He merely has to listen to himself, to the inner promptings that drive him or direct him to act upon something.

In cases of depression, low energy, or low self-esteem we can shower ourselves with vibrant colors like red, orange, yellow, and green. You will notice that they correspond to the root chakra, the sacral chakra, the solar plexus chakra, and the heart chakra. Those are the very chakras that need balancing so simply breathe in or meditate upon the corresponding color.

Add the color pink and you will have addressed issues on self-love. Love starts with self anyway so why not nurture and nourish yourself first? Get your energy back first!

The body has great intelligence. You only have to listen to it, to your feelings at that moment, and it will tell you where you are hurting, where you need to energize, to re-balance, to heal, to strengthen.

Consider this example: You are feeling tired and depleted. Your blood pressure seems low. You drag yourself through the day, with hardly any energy to get up from bed. You wish you could just stay in bed all day long.

Maybe that is exactly what you need – to stay in bed all day long. But what if you have work?

Although eating something sweet or having a strong jolt of java may give you that boost, you may just find that it is a temporary fix.

The real issues may lie underneath, and you may have to review where your life is at the moment. Perhaps you feel unloved. Perhaps you ate too much the night before or drank too much liquor – more than your mind and body can handle – and today you feel wasted. Perhaps you are coming down with a cold. Perhaps you are not happy at work, and you dread getting up. Your body worked in consonance with you, creating a convenient excuse not to have to work.

Perhaps there are issues that keep coming back to you, much as you keep setting them aside. Now you feel heavy, unattractive, unloved, low, depressed, lethargic, even ill.

That's the beauty of the body. It lets you know at any given moment. *We are a thinking, feeling species and our body is our best friend.*

Take this example for instance: We are barefoot and we step on a small piece of broken glass. Right away we feel that pain, and our body alerts its whole healing system protecting itself from further injury and intrusion.

Night and day the body protects us from harm. It is truly our best friend and ally. You may even be getting into small accidents because your mind is engaged elsewhere. It is always good to have presence of mind.

We are all warriors on earth and a slight slip may cost us our life or limb, our future, our well-being, and may even affect others who cross our path. They become the unwitting object of our anger or carelessness.

Conclusion

The Energizing, Healing Power of Color

Chromotherapy is a useful tool. It is an aid, a guide, an avenue towards healing. The real healer is YOUR SELF.

It probably follows that if you caused the illness upon yourself, then only you can heal that very disease. Disease has been called "dis-ease" for we lost that ease we originally had. When children become adults they get "adulterated". The freshness and innocence is often lost by arrogance, pride, or ego.

As energetic beings, children have such pure spirits. They are so fresh and inspiring for they have no fear. They only know possibilities. They make the rules as they go along.

On our part, we adults make too many rules and impose too many strict measures upon ourselves. No wonder we can't breathe! Then we become hesitant and fearful, and we lose strength, courage, and determination. And we wonder why our health suffers and we contract disease. We have lost that "ease".

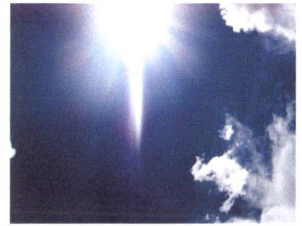

Let us use *color therapy* as a handy, happy, and friendly tool. When we are feeling down, we can simply follow our first instincts and wear a color or look at a color that energizes us. We have to listen to ourselves, that inner physician, who really knows what's going on with our bodies. It is he who has first access to our hearts, minds, bodies, and spirits.

Do what resonates well with your spirit. If you are a meditator then heal yourself with the best colors that lift your spirit.

If you are not a meditator then go to an art gallery that has happy, positive, and uplifting paintings and draw upon a color that fascinates you.

Or maybe, paint your own artwork in the colors that appeal to you at that moment! Be childlike in your mind's adventure!

If you enjoy shopping and you have the funds to sustain such, then lift your spirits by purchasing items whose colors make you happy.

It's time to feel good again! Only you can give yourself the happiness you so need. Who knows you more than you? Why not start with self and please self for a change?

Nurture that self and give it the joy it needs, without guilt, and just enjoy being yourself. When you are happy, your whole self would glow... You yourself will exhibit all the colors of the rainbow, and people will be attracted to your spirit!

That very simple act of cultivating love for self in all its entirety will be the most healing act of all. On a deeper level, you know yourself. You know what's good for you. You get sick when you go against the grain and do something else. You betray yourself, your instincts, and your emotions.

You become sick when you are unhappy. You already carry all the colors of the rainbow in your heart. All that you need is right in your heart. If you are to meditate upon a color, then do so from your heart. Your heart will tell you the colors that you lack. Acknowledge the wisdom of your heart and you will surely heal!

Your heart knows everything about you. You simply have to listen to its wisdom. Follow your heart. It knows what's best for you. Take courage. The power of healing is within you.

Become trusting and childlike again. Trust that inner child in you that loves to play, to be happy, to experiment, to explore, to rest, to dream.

Children don't even care what colors they wear. They don't even care if their colors match. They just want to play. They instinctively know what feels good, what feels right, and they go right into it. No ifs and buts.

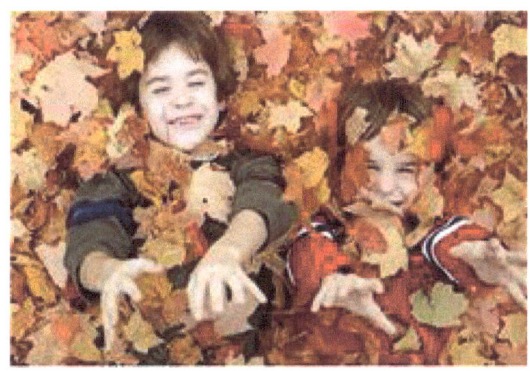

But we adults always think they look funny when their colors don't match. Precisely! In a child's world what fun is there when everything matches and there's no individuality?

Become at ease again. Make life a picnic once again! Have more fun, more joy, more freedom, less rules, no scoring for that is boring.

Become light of spirit, and you will discover in that very lightness that you carry all the colors of the rainbow. Your light will shine

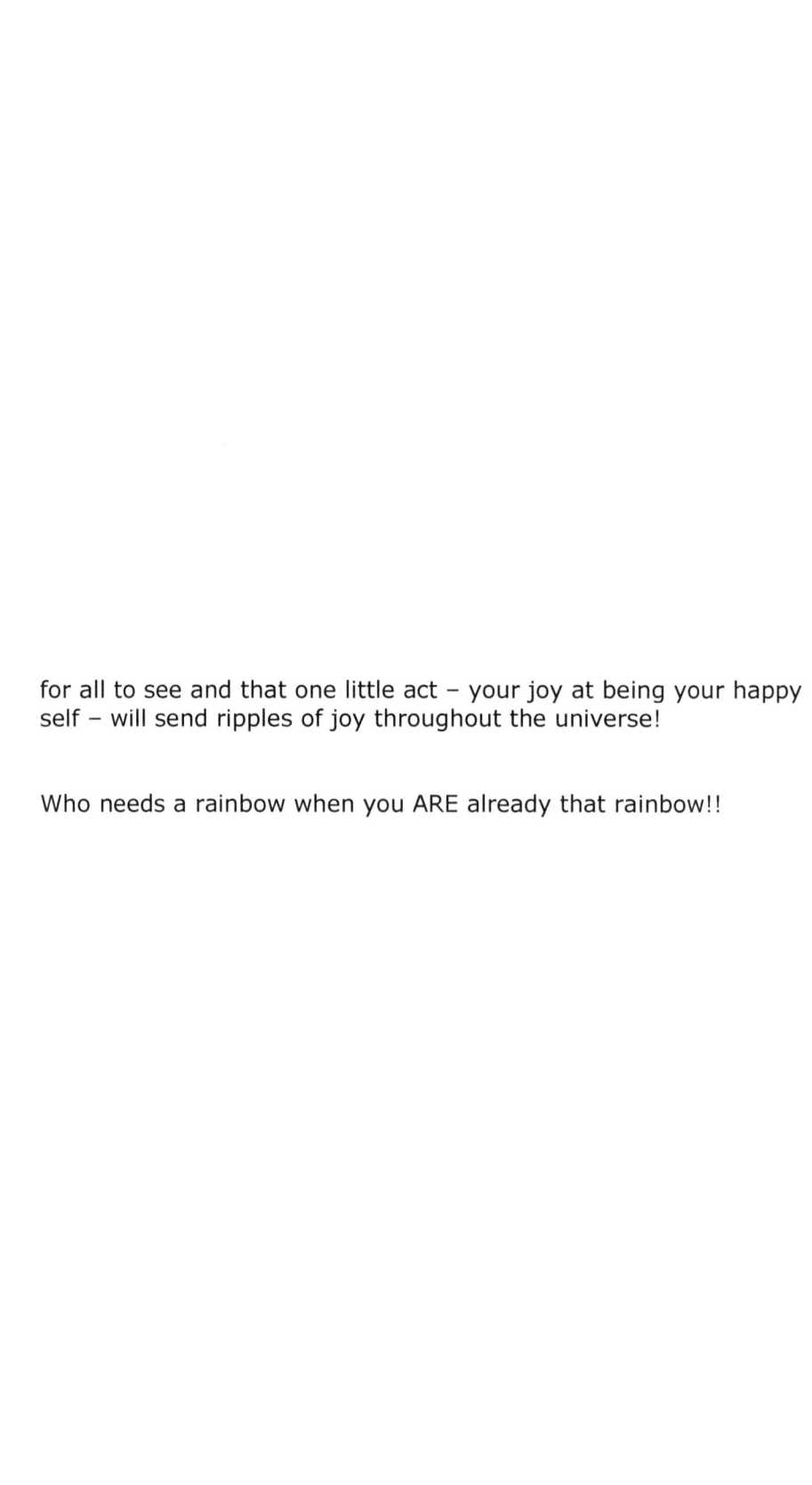

for all to see and that one little act – your joy at being your happy self – will send ripples of joy throughout the universe!

Who needs a rainbow when you ARE already that rainbow!!